# Waikiki Jogger

# Honolulu - a Jogger's Paradise

# Waikiki Jogger
## 21 Routes for Runners

## Dennis M Keating

## Maps & Illustrations
## Dennis M Keating

### DEDICATION

## To all the Joggers in Honolulu

This book, its maps and information
are the property of their creator
The Honolulu Guy,
Dennis M Keating

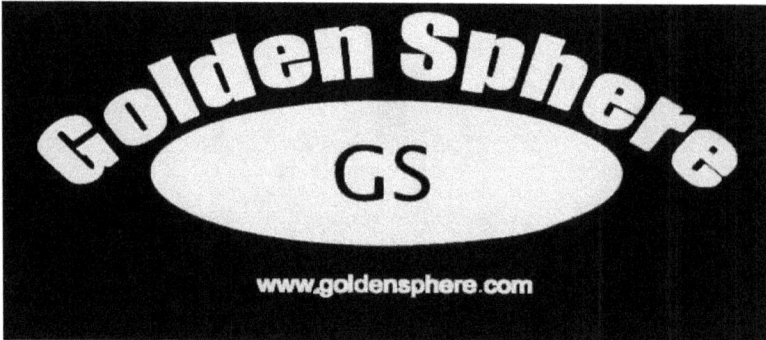

Golden Sphere
GS
www.goldensphere.com

# Waikiki Jogger

**Waikiki Jogger** is a guide for Honolulu locals and Waikiki visitors who enjoy running or taking walks.

This book features twenty-one jogging maps. Each map offers one or more measured jogging routes. The order of the maps is for the convenience of first-time visitors, with the base routes starting and finishing in Waikiki. Naturally, local runners who are familiar with the areas will start their runs wherever they prefer. The book provides routes that connect to the base routes for runners who are eager to expand their confines and combine their jogging experience with exploration of bits of Honolulu's beautiful scenery.

Waikiki is ideally situated between Honolulu's two major park, Kapiolani Park on the Diamond Head side and Ala Moana Park on the downtown side. Both parks front the ocean and are highly popular with local residents. The jogging routes in this book are designed to limit the number of cross streets runners may encounter. The shortest route is a little more than a quarter of a mile and the longest is sixteen miles.

# Honolulu's Weather

Thanks to our Tradewinds and tropical location we enjoy ideal jogging weather all year long. There is no serious rainy season. While rain is a daily thing in the mountains, Waikiki experiences very limited rainfall. Our nickname for this gentle rain is pineapple juice.

| Month | High/Low(°F) | High/Low (°C) |
|---|---|---|
| January | 78°/71° | 26°/21° |
| February | 77°/ 71° | 25°/21° |
| March | 77°/ 71° | 25°/21° |
| April | 79°/ 72° | 26°/22° |
| May | 81°/ 74° | 27°/23° |
| June | 82°/ 75° | 27°/23° |
| July | 83°/ 76° | 28°/24° |
| August | 84°/ 77° | 29°/25° |
| September | 84°/ 77° | 29°/25° |
| October | 83°/ 76° | 28°/24° |
| November | 81°/ 74° | 27°/23° |
| December | 79°/ 72° | 26°/22° |

These rounded estimates are based on government data.

# Waikiki's Sunrise/Sunset Times

## These estimates for the first day of the month

| Month | Sunrise | Sunset |
|-------|---------|--------|
| January | 7:10 | 6:00 |
| February | 7:10 | 6:20 |
| March | 6:50 | 6:35 |
| April | 6:25 | 6:45 |
| May | 6:00 | 6:55 |
| June | 5:50 | 7:10 |
| July | 5:50 | 7:15 |
| August | 6:05 | 7:10 |
| September | 6:15 | 6:45 |
| October | 6:25 | 6:15 |
| November | 6:35 | 5:55 |
| December | 6:55 | 5:45 |

Hawaii is closer to the equator than the other 49 states, so our daylight periods are longer in the winter months and shorter in the summer months.

# #1064, The Wall & the Rainbow

For Waikiki visitors, we suggest one of three optional starting points.
The first starting point is the **#1064 fire hydrant,** in the heart of Waikiki.

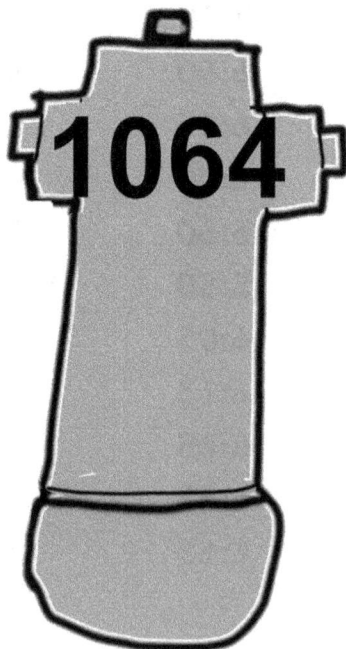

**1064**

**Good old # 1064** is on Kalakaua Avenue in front of the **Royal Hawaiian Shopping Center,** directly across from Seaside Avenue.

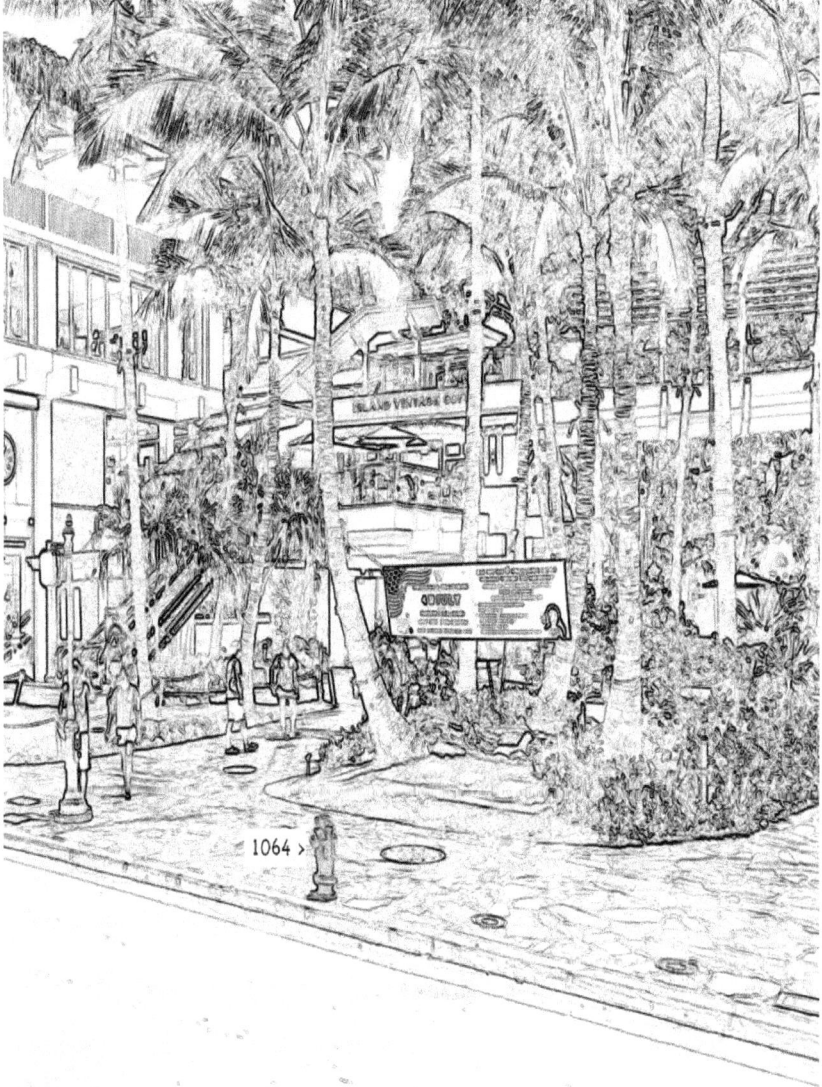

The second starting point, **The Wall,** is on the Diamond Head end of Waikiki beach. Joggers can start in front of the concrete pier that is part of **The Wall.** This pier faces Kalakaua Avenue and is directly across from Kapahulu Avenue.

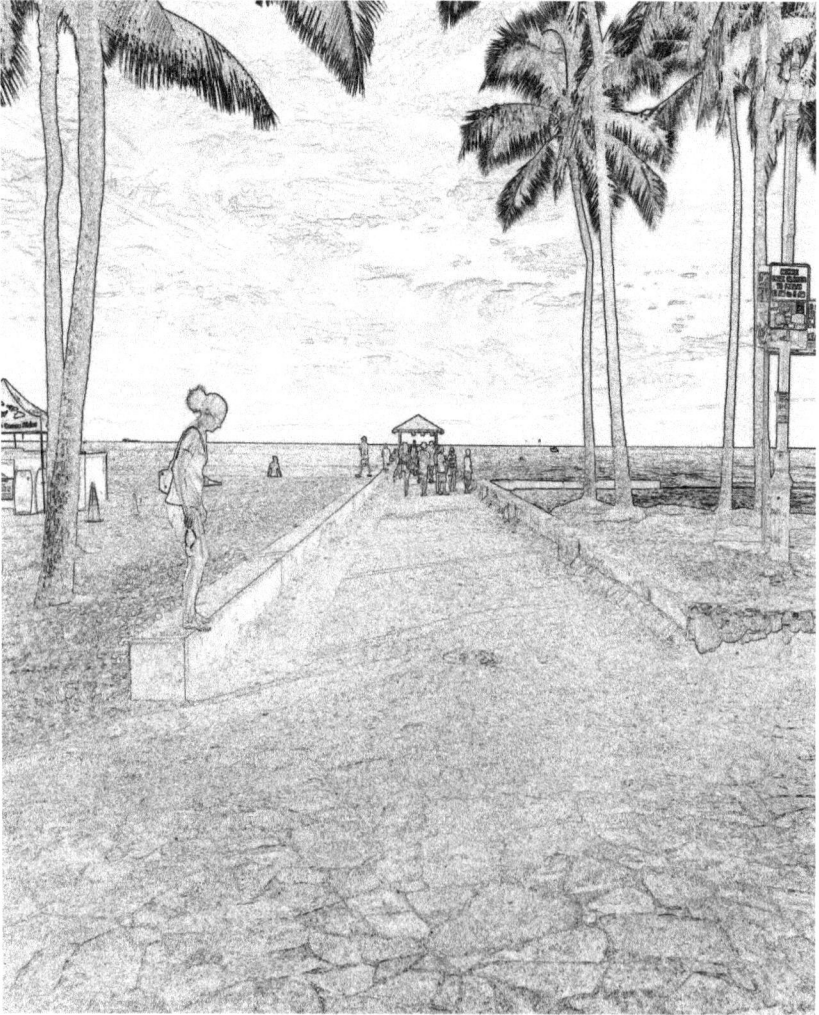

The third starting point we call, Rainbow. It's under the Rainbow Tower mural of the Hilton Hawaiian Village. It is roughly in the middle of the **Strolling Route** where Beachwalk ends, and the Lagoon path begins.

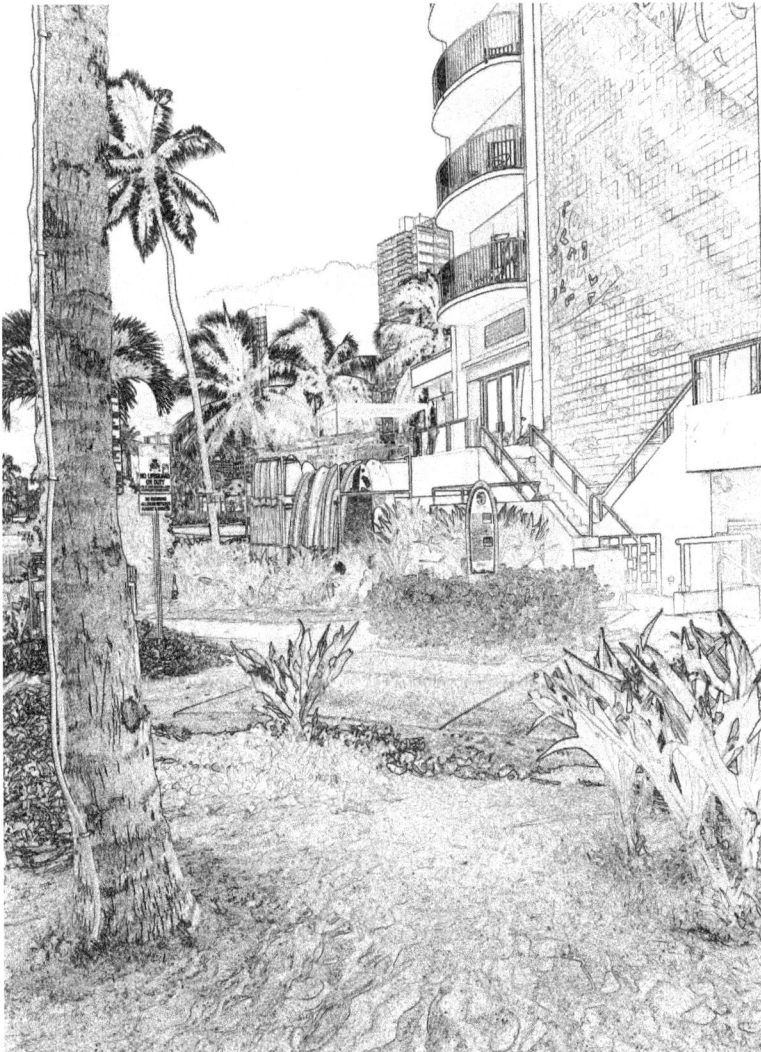

## ACKNOWLEDGMENTS

To all my old jogging buddies and especially my wife, who has outrun me in every race we have ever joined together including the annual Honolulu Marathon.

\* \* \*

## Dennis M Keating
### is a retired marathon
### runner and fun jogger

Keating took up jogging in 1970. Maybe that wasn't before country became country, but it was before Nike became Nike and before Honolulu hosted its first marathon.

Since that time Keating has jogged virtually all over the world from Moscow to Manila, Brussels to Bangkok, and Cork to Chicago. He has not found a more suitable place to jog than in Honolulu. That's one of the main reasons he retired in Waikiki.

Now, he takes walks, goes for coffee or beer in Waikiki and enjoys writing books.

He has two jogging recommendations. The first concerns personal hydration. When running long distances, drink a sufficient amount of water. While this book highlights numerous water fountains, he cautions they are not always functioning properly.

His second recommendation is to run with a buddy. This is for camaraderie, support and safety.

# Listing of Routes

We consider the measurements in this book to be guidelines rather than absolutes, as individual runners have slight difference in their ways of rounding corners and staying to the left, middle or right. Each route was walked and measured multiple times with a surveyor measuring wheel. When results differed, the routes were remeasured a third or fourth time. The results were then compared with distances calculated by internet websites. We believe all the measures are accurate. If you feel one is out of whack, please contact the author at lostpuka@gmail.com

# Diamond Head Direction Routes

# The Strip

## 1064 > The Wall
### The Base Run: Diamond Head Direction

|  | Miles | Kilometers |
|---|---|---|
| **One Way** | | |
| 1064 > The Wall | .6 | 1.0 |
| | | |
| **Round Trip Start/Finish** | | |
| @ 1064 | 1.3 | 2.0 |
| @ Rainbow | 3.3 | 5.3 |

**Scene:** Waikiki's main drag

**Start:** 1064

**Return Point:** Sidewalk fronting The Wall

**Water Fountain:** Yes

**Restrooms:** Yes

**Cross Streets:** None

Link Runs
@ 1064: Saratoga & By the sea, not!
@ The Wall: Crown, Cheetah, Racetrack & Daily Double

Comment: Be prepared to zigzag around strolling tourists. The Wall, a Waikiki fixture, starts at the pier across from Kapahulu Avenue. To local surfers this area is known as Walls.

# The Strip
## 1064 > The Wall

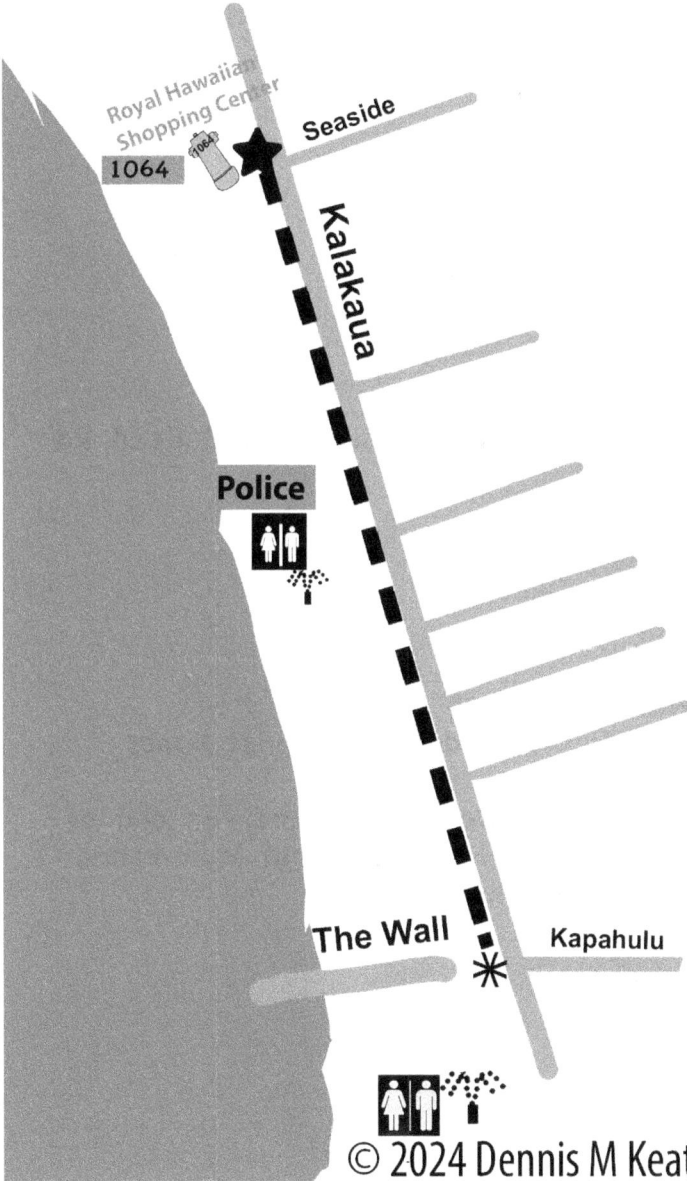

Royal Hawaiian
Shopping Center

1064

Seaside

Kalakaua

Police

The Wall

Kapahulu

© 2024 Dennis M Keating

# Crown
## The Wall > Poni Moi Road

|  | Miles | Kilometers |
|---|---|---|
| **One Way** | | |
| The Wall > Poni Moi | .9 | 1.4 |
| | | |
| **Round Trip Start/Finish** | | |
| @ Walls | 1.8 | 2.8 |
| @ 1064 | 3.0 | 4.8 |
| @ Rainbow | 5.0 | 8.1 |

Scene: Park setting
Start: The Wall
Return Point: Poni Moi Rd & Diamond Head Rd

Water Fountain: Yes
Restroom: Yes
Cross Streets: Two

Link Runs
@ The Wall: The Strip
@ Poni Moi & Diamond Head Roads: Honor

Comment: Poni Moi Road is at the far end of Kapiolani Park. In Hawaiian, Poni Moi means coronation or crown.

# Crown

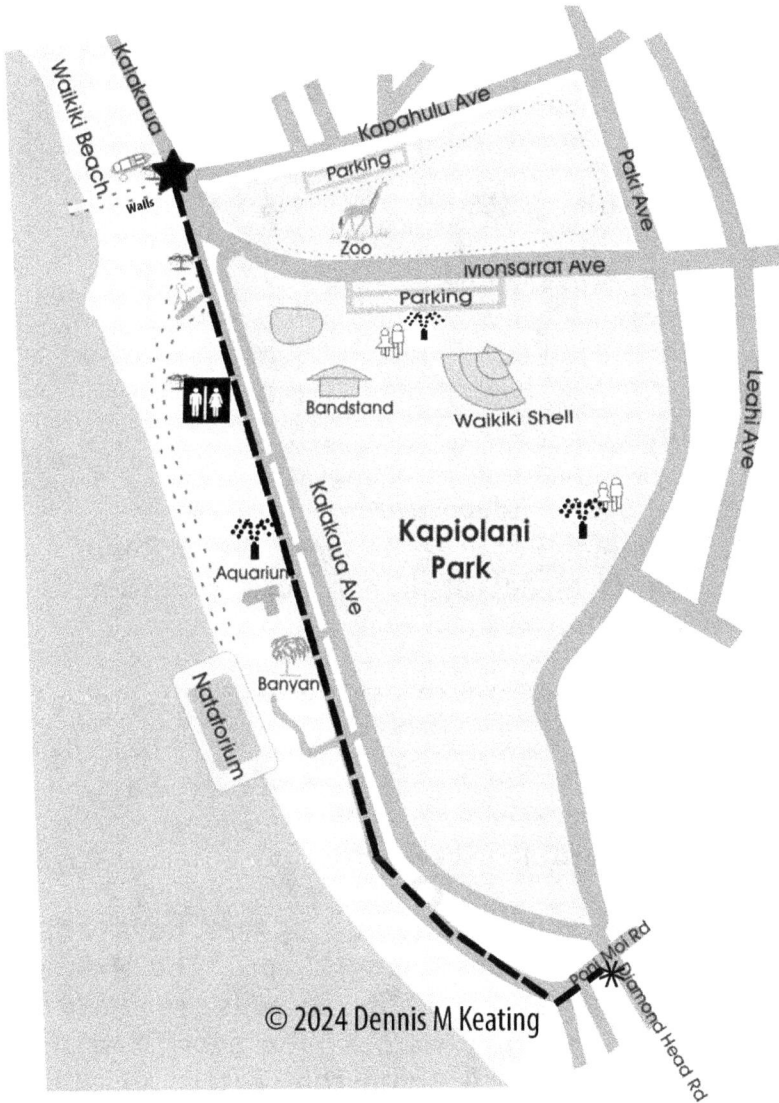

Waikiki Beach.

Kalakaua

Kapahulu Ave

Parking

Walls

Zoo

Monsarrat Ave

Paki Ave

Parking

Bandstand

Waikiki Shell

Leahi Ave

Kalakaua Ave

Kapiolani Park

Aquarium

Natatorium

Banyan

Pau Moi Rd

Diamond Head Rd

© 2024 Dennis M Keating

# Honor
## Poni Moi Road >Triangle Water Fountain at Operation Red Wings Medal of Honor Park

| | Miles | Kilometers |
|---|---|---|
| One Way | | |
| Poni Moi > | | |
| Water Fountain | 1.6 | 2.6 |
| | | |
| Round Trip Start/Finish | | |
| @ Poni Moi | 3.2 | 5.1 |
| @ Walls | 5.0 | 8.0 |
| @ 1064 | 6.2 | 10.0 |
| @ Rainbow | 8.0 | 12.9 |

Scene: An uphill adventure
Start: Poni Moi Road at Diamond Head Road
Return Point: Medal of Honor Park fountain
Water Fountain: Yes
Restroom: No
Cross Streets: Six

Link Runs
@ Poni Moi: Crown
@ Water Fountain: Gas Station

Comment: For decades, local joggers have called this rest point "The Triangle" or "The Triangle water fountain." In 2008, it was renamed to honor the US military heroes who sacrificed their lives at the 2005 Afghanistan Battle of Abbas Ghar.
On older maps this park is called Fort Ruger Park.

# Honor

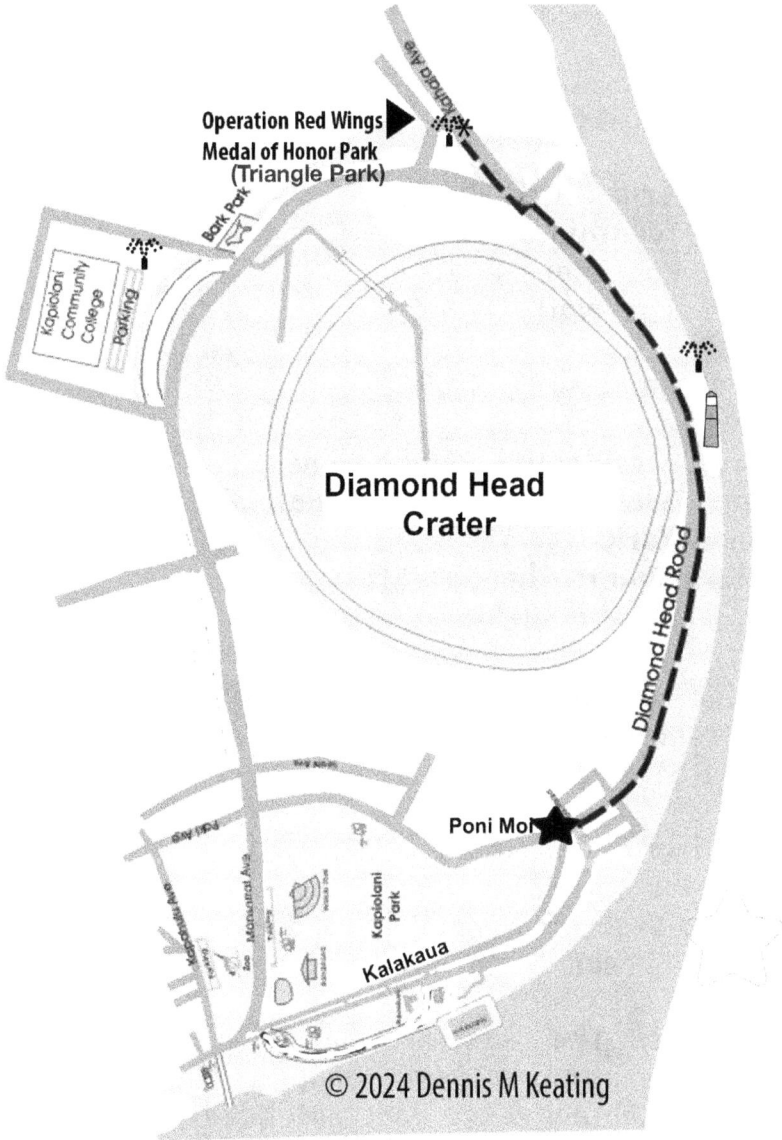

**Operation Red Wings Medal of Honor Park (Triangle Park)**

Kapiolani Community College

Parking

Bark Park

Diamond Head Crater

Diamond Head Road

Poni Moi

Kapiolani Park

Kalakaua

© 2024 Dennis M Keating

# Gas Station
## Water Fountain > Gas Station

|  | Miles | Kilometers |
|---|---|---|
| One Way |  |  |
| Fountain> Gas Station | 2.0 | 3.3 |
| | | |
| **Round Trip Start/Finish** | | |
| @ Fountain | 4.0 | 6.6 |
| @ Poni Moi | 7.3 | 11.7 |
| @ The Wall | 9.0 | 14.6 |
| @ 1064 | 10.3 | 16.6 |
| @ Rainbow | 11.9 | 19.1 |

Scene: Residential neighborhood.
Start: Water fountain @ Medal of Honor Park
Return Point: The Gas Station at Kalaniana'ole Highway

Water Fountain: Yes
Restroom: No
Cross Streets: Twelve

Link Runs
@ Water Fountain: Honor
@ Gas Station: None. You're done.
Take a break & go back the way you came.

Comment: The Gas Station is a local jogger landmark, and a key Honolulu Marathon turn point. Kahala Avenue does not have sidewalks, so joggers must run along the edge of the street.

# Gas Station

Gas Station ▶ ✳

Kealaolu

Kahala

◀ Waikiki

Operation
Red Wings
Medal of Honor
Park (Triangle Park)

Kahala Ave

© 2024 Dennis M Keating

# Cheetah
## Loop the Zoo

| | Miles | Kilometers |
|---|---|---|
| Zoo Loop | 1.1 | 1.8 |
| | | |
| Round Trip Start/Finish | | |
| @ 1064 | 2.4 | 3.9 |
| @ Rainbow | 3.2 | 5.1 |

Scene: Perimeter of the Honolulu Zoo
Start: Front of Zoo across from The Wall
Return Point: None. A loop run

Water Fountain: No
Restroom: No
Cross Streets: None

Link Runs
@ Front of Zoo: The Strip,
Racetrack, Daily Double

Comment: While this run loops the zoo, the bushes and fence shield the animals except for an occasional giraffe head. Want a role model? Try the cheetah, the fastest animal in the world. Cheetahs can run a mile a minute.

# Cheetah

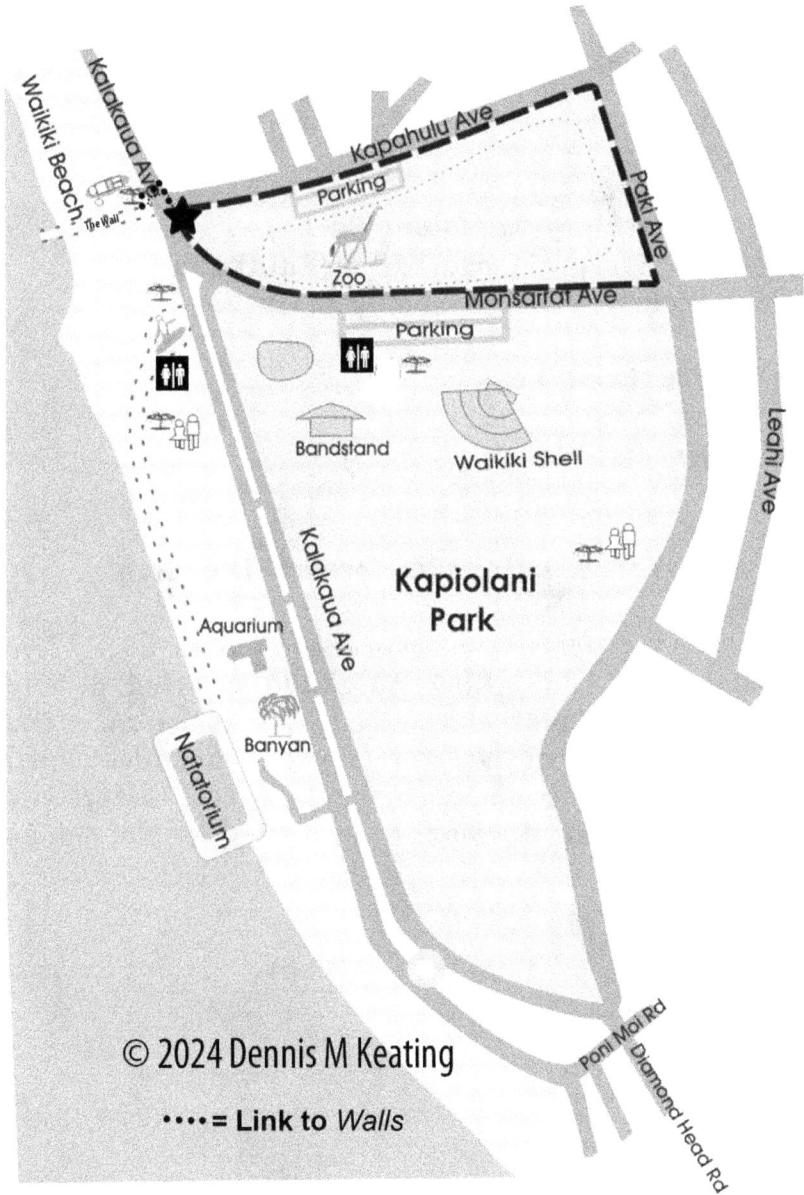

Waikiki Beach

Kalakaua Ave

Kapahulu Ave

Paki Ave

Parking

The Wail

Zoo

Monsarrat Ave

Parking

Leahi Ave

Bandstand

Waikiki Shell

Kapiolani
Park

Aquarium

Kalakaua Ave

Banyan

Natatorium

© 2024 Dennis M Keating

•••• = **Link to** *Walls*

Poni Moi Rd

Diamond Head Rd

# Racetrack
## Kapiolani Park Loop

|              | Miles | Kilometers |
|--------------|-------|------------|
| Park Loop    | 1.5   | 2.5        |

Round Trip Start/Finish
| @ 1064    | 2.8 | 4.5 |
|-----------|-----|-----|
| @ Rainbow | 3.6 | 5.7 |

Scene: Encircling Kapiolani Park
Start: Corner of Monsarrat & Kalakaua
Return Point: None. A loop run

Water Fountain: Yes
Restroom: Yes
Cross Streets: None

Link Runs
@ Monsarrat & Kalakaua Corner: The Strip,
Cheetah

Comment: In 1883, King Kalakaua created a mile long horse racetrack at this location. The racetrack was active for several decades until someone decided an open park would offer the public healthier options than losing their money on the ponies.

# Racetrack

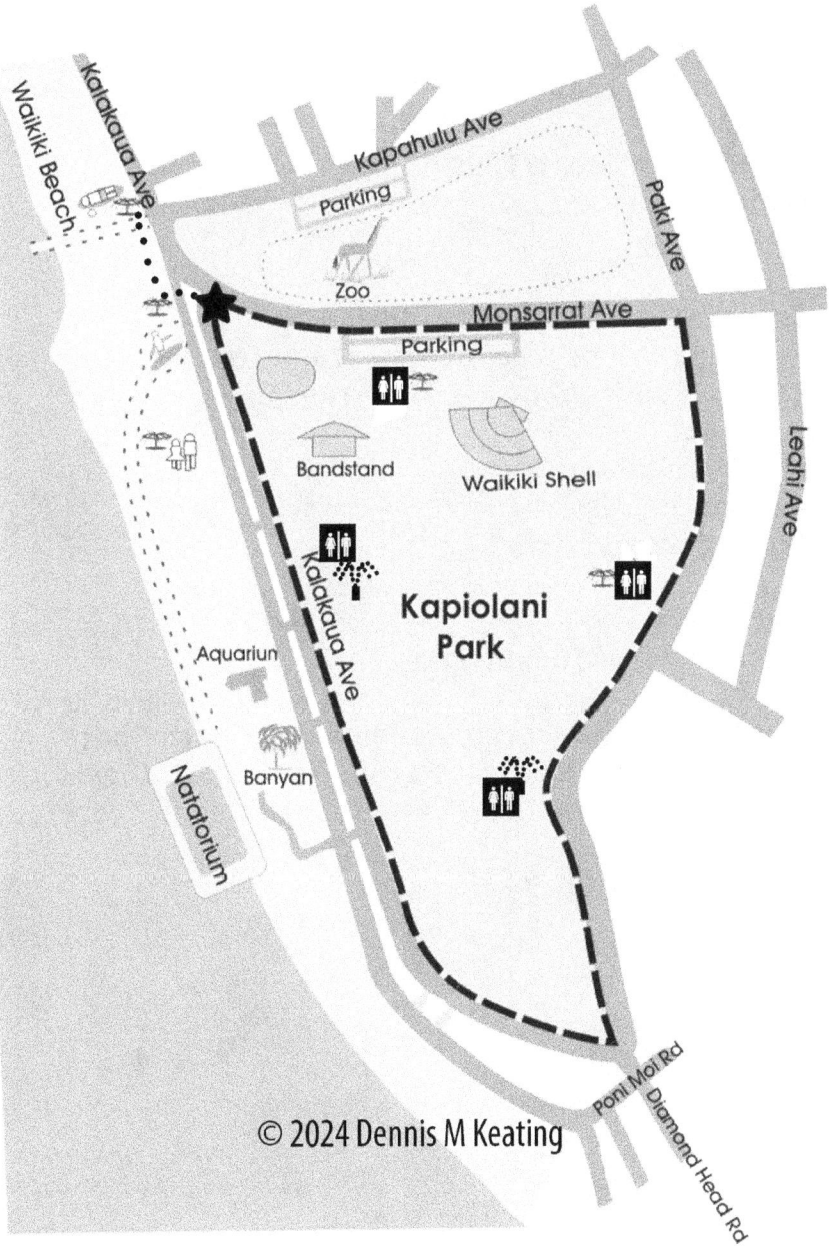

© 2024 Dennis M Keating

# Daily Double
## Kapiolani Park & Zoo Loops

|  | Miles | Kilometers |
|---|---|---|
| One Combo Loop | 2.1 | 3.4 |

Round Trip Start/Finish

| | Miles | Kilometers |
|---|---|---|
| @ 1064 | 3.4 | 5.4 |
| @ Rainbow | 4.2 | 6.7 |

Scene: A zoo and park combo
Start: Front of zoo across from The Wall
Return Point: None. A loop run

Water Fountain: Yes
Restroom: Yes
Cross Streets: Two

Link Runs
@ The Wall: The Strip

Comment: This area is popular with both visitors and locals. Family outings, sports activities, festivals, concerts and picnics are the norm.

# Daily Double

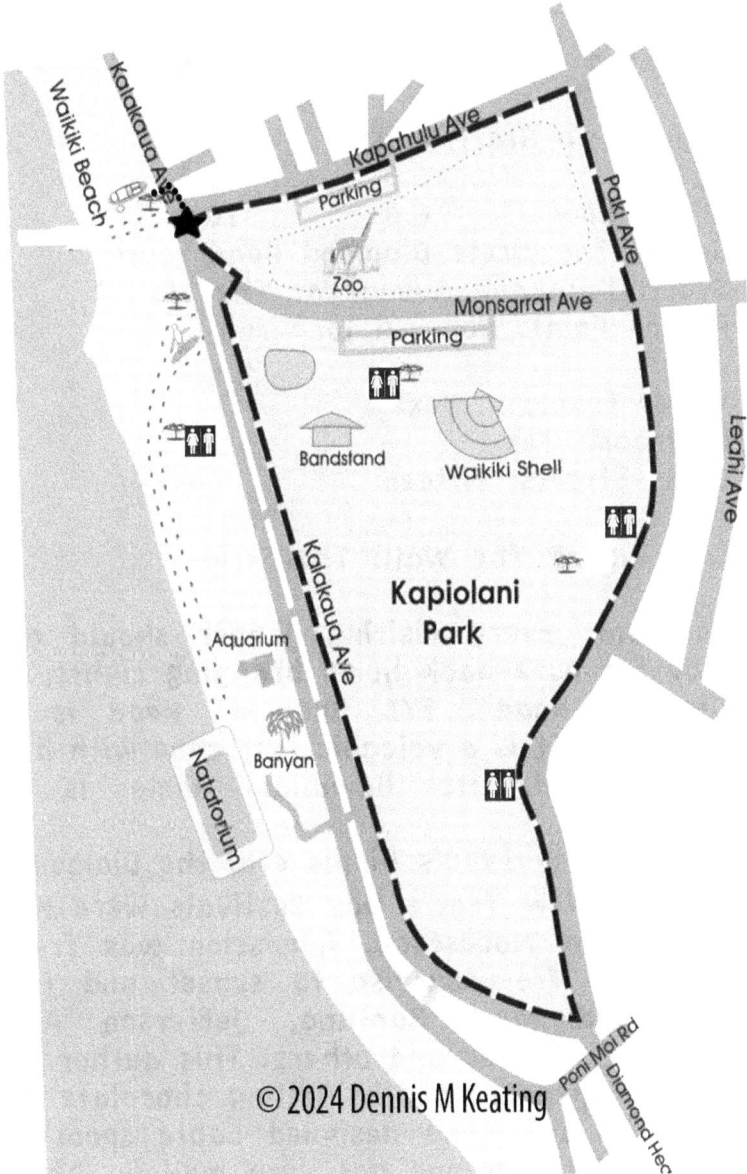

© 2024 Dennis M Keating

# The Jewel
## Diamond Head Loop
## with Triangle Park

|  | Miles | Kilometers |
|---|---|---|
| One Loop | 4.7 | 7.6 |

Round Trip Start/Finish

|  | Miles | Kilometers |
|---|---|---|
| @ 1064 | 6.0 | 9.6 |
| @ Rainbow | 6.6 | 10.6 |

Scene: The circle Diamond Head route
Start: Kalakaua Avenue at The Wall
Return Point: None. A loop run

Water Fountain: Yes
Restroom: Yes
Cross Streets: Fifteen

Link Run @ The Wall: The Strip

Comment: Every visiting jogger should do this loop for pure back home bragging rights, "I ran Diamond Head". FYI, Diamond Head is not a mountain. It is a volcanic tuff cone with a crater inside; and, its Hawaiian name is Leahi.

In the early 1970's Hippie era, the Diamond Head Crater's New Year's Day Festivals were Hawaii's answer to Woodstock. Admission was free. The fest ran from sunrise to sunset and featured Fleetwood Mac, Santana, Jefferson Airplane, Cecilio & Kapono and others. This author and his friends operated booths selling chocolate covered bananas and hand designed cable spool tables. Meanwhile everyone got very mellow. Ah! Those were the days my friend. Those were the days.

# The Jewel

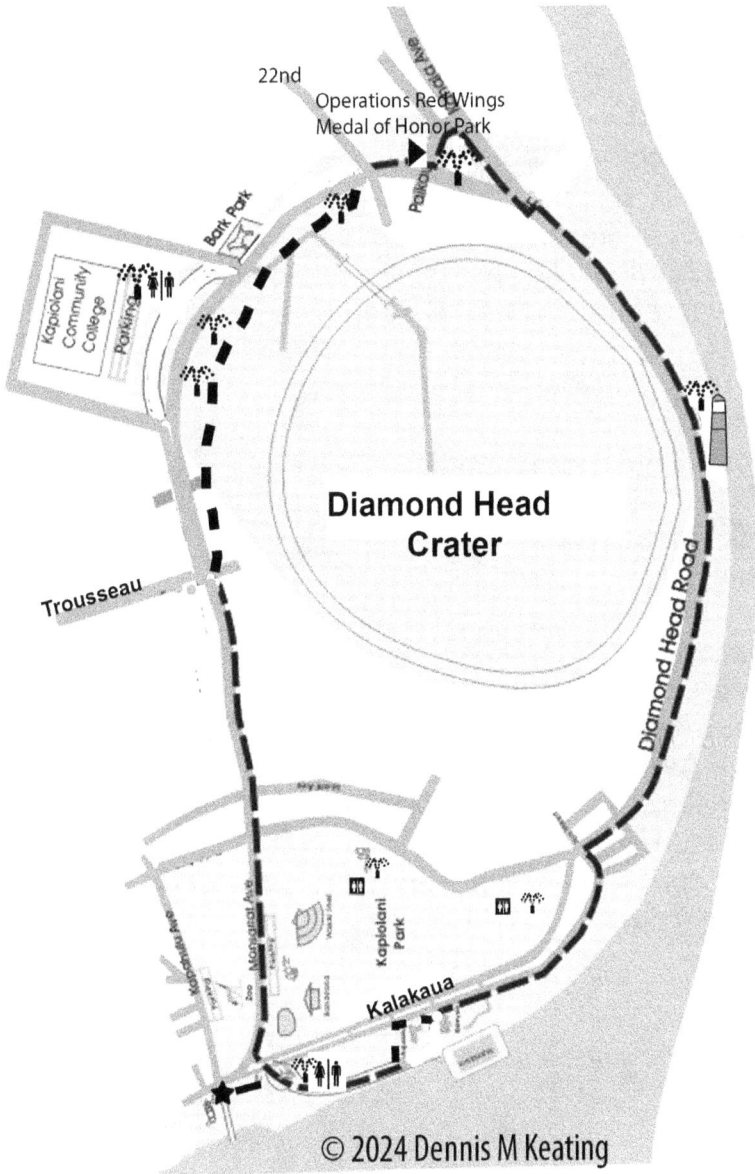

22nd

Operations Red Wings
Medal of Honor Park

Bork Park

Kapiolani
Community
College

Parking

Pokai Ave

Trousseau

**Diamond Head Crater**

Diamond Head Road

Kapiolani Ave

Monsarrat Ave

Kapiolani Park

Kalakaua

© 2024 Dennis M Keating

17

# Kama'aina Discount Route
## Diamond Head with Triangle Loop
### (Favored by Locals)

|  | Miles | Kilometers |
|---|---|---|
| One Loop: | 4.0 | 6.5 |

Scene: A more snug Diamond Head route.
Start/Finish: Corner of Paki & Monsarrat
Return Point: None. A loop run

Water Fountain: Yes
Restroom: Yes
Cross Streets: Thirteen

Link Runs
None

Comment: This shorter Diamond Head loop is favored by local joggers. This is not because we are lazy (well, most of us), but rather, because Paki Avenue offers free parking places with the additional perk of allowing the jogger to avoid the madness of Waikiki.
This route does not directly connect with the other routes in this book.

# Kama'aina Discount Route

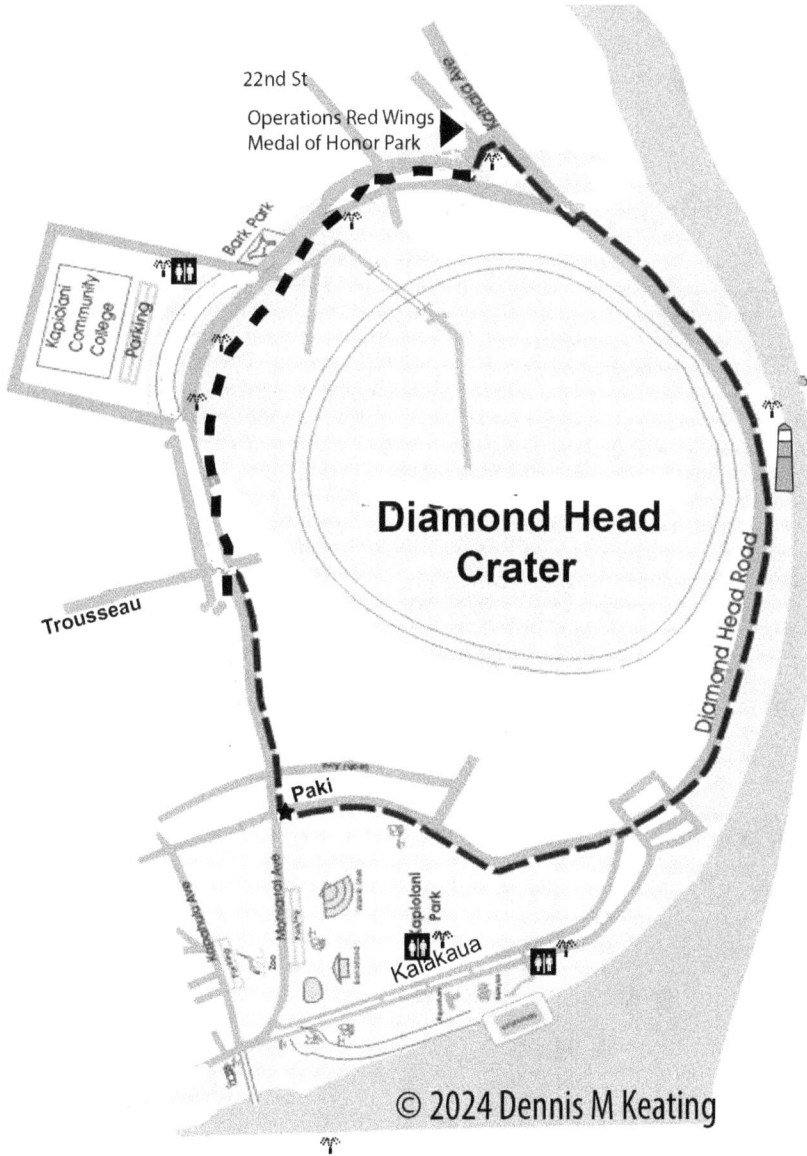

22nd St

Operations Red Wings
Medal of Honor Park

Diamond Head Crater

Kapiolani Community College

Parking

Bark Park

Trousseau

Paki

Kapiolani Park

Kalakaua

Kalakaua Ave

Monsarrat Ave

Diamond Head Road

© 2024 Dennis M Keating

# Mauka (Mountain) Direction Routes

# Seaside, by the sea. . . not!
## 1064 > Ala Wai Canal
## The Base Run: Mountain Direction

|  | Miles | Kilometers |
|---|---|---|
| One Way | .3 | .5 |

Round Trip Start/Finish
| | | |
|---|---|---|
| @ 1064 | .6 | .9 |
| @ Walls | 1.8 | 2.9 |
| @ Rainbow | 2.6 | 4.2 |

Scene: Waikiki's Seaside Avenue, a side street
Start: 1064
Return Point: Sidewalk @ the Ala Wai Canal

Water Fountain: No
Restroom: No
Cross Streets: Three

Link Runs
@ 1064: Saratoga & The Strip

Comment: This is an unglamorous connector run. Seaside Avenue? Don't let the street name fool you. As one old timer said, "You ain't not never, no way, no how gonna see the sea from Seaside Avenue."

# Seaside, by the sea. . . not!

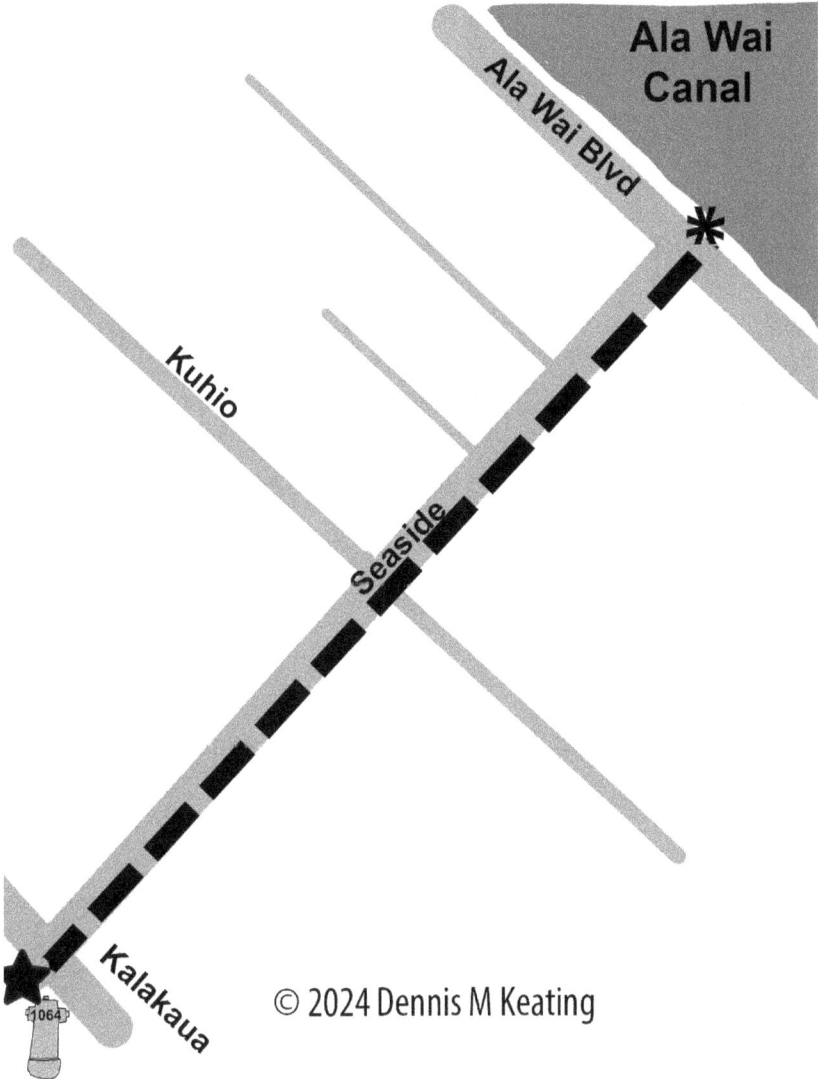

Ala Wai Canal

Ala Wai Blvd

Kuhio

Seaside

Kalakaua

1064

© 2024 Dennis M Keating

# Dig it
## Ala Wai Canal Strip

|  | Miles | Kilometers |
|---|---|---|
| One Full Length | 1.4 | 2.3 |
| Up & Back | 2.9 | 4.7 |

Round Trip Start/Finish

|  | Miles | Kilometers |
|---|---|---|
| @ 1064 | 3.4 | 5.5 |
| @ Walls | 4.7 | 7.5 |
| @ Rainbow | 4.9 | 7.9 |

Scene: Ala Wai Canal with a Koʻolau mountain view
Start & Finish: Ala Wai Canal at Seaside Ave
Two Return Points: Downtown side, McCully Ave; Diamond Head side, Kapahulu Avenue

Water Fountain: No
Public Restroom: No
Cross Streets: None

Link Run
@ Ala Wai Blvd & Seaside: By the sea, not!

Comment: The Hawaii Territorial Government authorized the digging of the Ala Wai Canal in the 1920's, in order to catch the water flowing into Waikiki from the Koʻolau mountains.

# Dig it

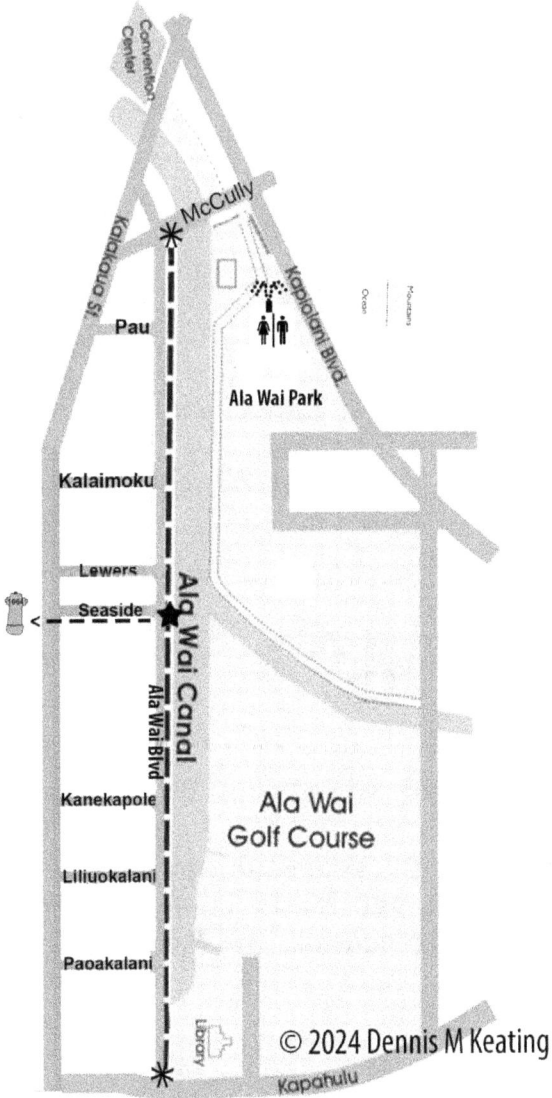

# Fore!
## Ala Wai Canal Loop

|  | Miles | Kilometers |
|---|---|---|
| One Loop | 3.5 | 5.7 |

| Round Trip Start/Finish | | |
|---|---|---|
| @ 1064 | 4.1 | 6.6 |
| @ Walls | 5.3 | 8.6 |
| @ Rainbow | 5.6 | 9.0 |

Scene: The Ala Wai Canal, the Ala Wai Park and the Ala Wai Golf Course.
Start: Ala Wai Canal at Seaside Avenue
Return Point: None. A loop run

Water Fountain: Yes
Public Restroom: Yes
Cross Streets: None

Link Run
@ Ala Wai Blvd & Seaside: By the sea, not!

Comment: The 90-year-old Ala Wai Golf Course is open to the public. It is one of the few affordable golf courses on Oahu.

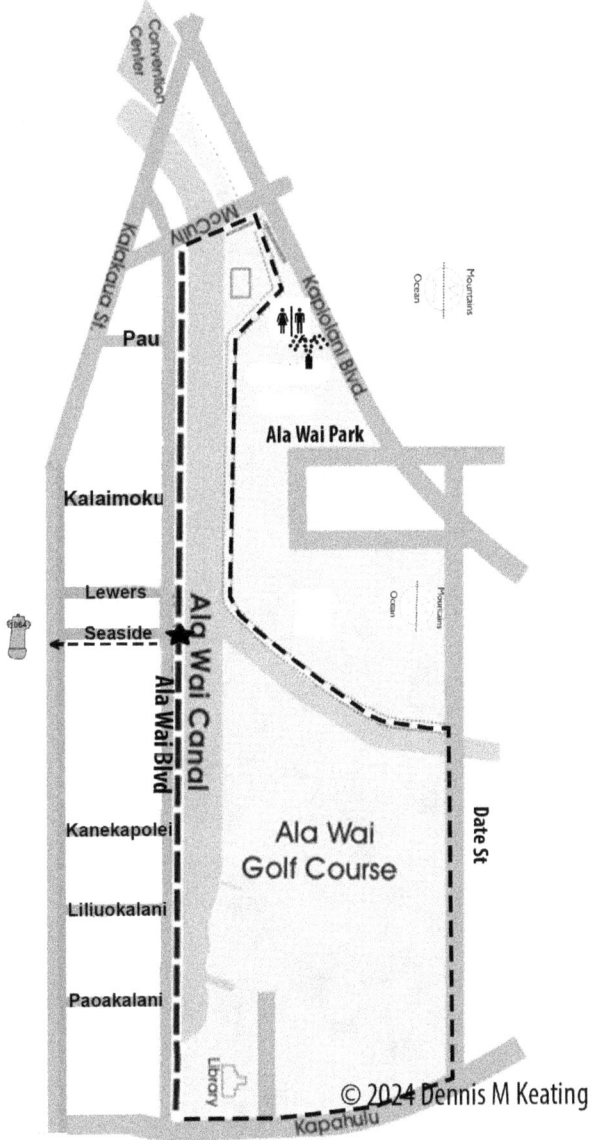

Fore!

# Downtown Direction Routes

# Saratoga
## 1064 > Saratoga
## The Base Run: Downtown Direction

|  | Miles | Kilometers |
|---|---|---|
| One Way | .6 | .9 |

Round Trip Start/Finish

| | Miles | Kilometers |
|---|---|---|
| @ 1064 | 1.2 | 1.9 |
| @ Walls | 2.4 | 3.9 |
| @ Rainbow | 3.2 | 5.1 |

Scene: Waikiki's main drag plus a long dog leg
Start: 1064
Return Point: Fort DeRussy Beachwalk

Water Fountain: Yes
Restroom: Yes (At end)
Cross Streets: Four

Link Runs
@ 1064: The Strip & By the sea, not!
@ Beachwalk: Beachwalk & Warrior

Comment: The name Saratoga comes from a bathhouse that stood in this locale in the early 1900's. Back in the day, Saratoga Springs, New York was well known for its mineral spring. I guess the owner felt a New York name would sound exotic in Hawaii.

# Saratoga

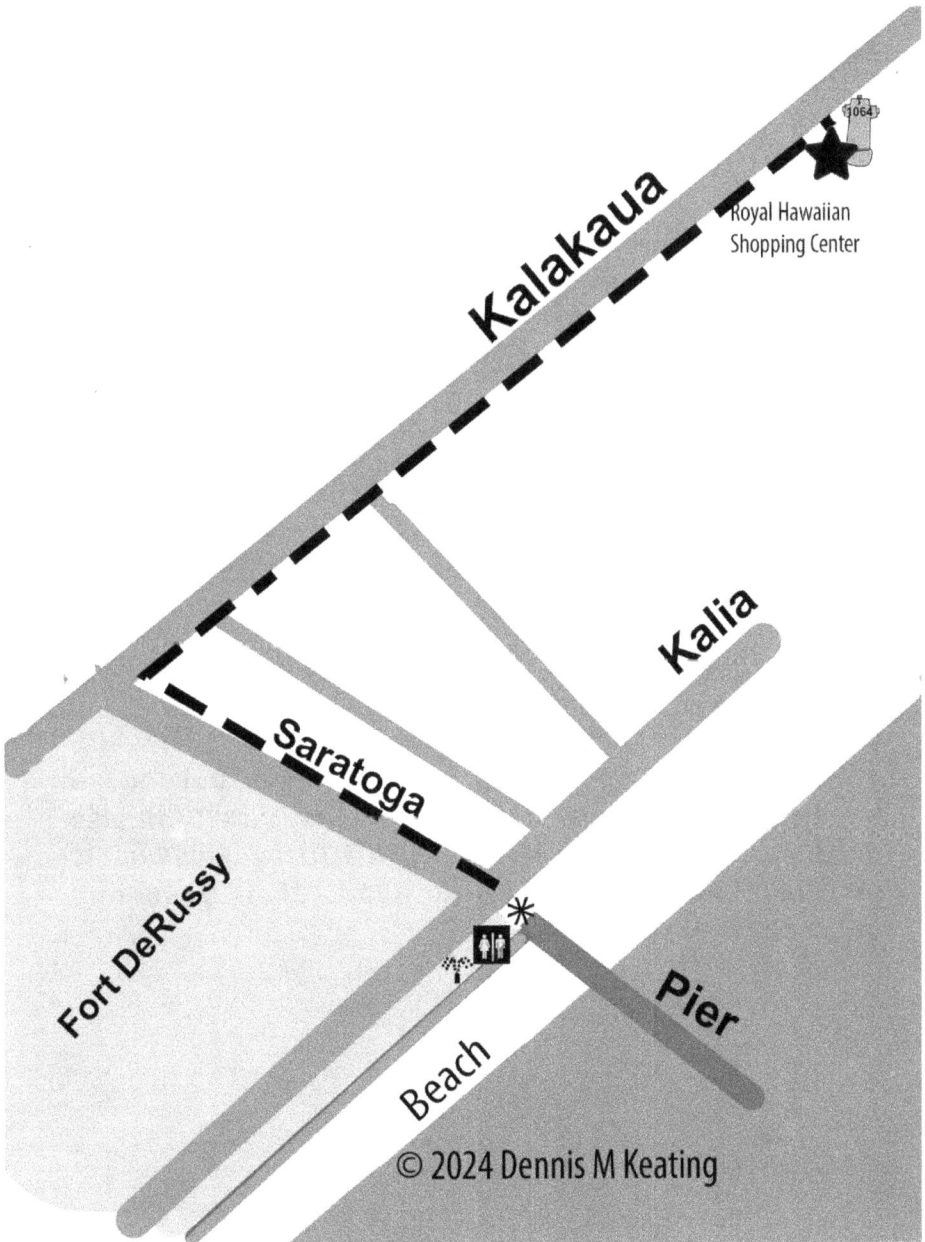

Kalakaua

Royal Hawaiian
Shopping Center

Kalia

Saratoga

Fort DeRussy

Pier

Beach

© 2024 Dennis M Keating

# Warrior
## Fort DeRussy Loop

|  | Miles | Kilometers |
|---|---|---|
| Park Loop | 1.1 | 1.8 |

Round trip Start & Finish
| @ 1064 | 2.3 | 3.7 |
|---|---|---|
| @ Walls | 3.5 | 5.7 |
| @ Rainbow | 2.1 | 3.4 |

Scene: Park setting
Start: Corner of Saratoga & Kalia
Return Point: None. A loop run

Water Fountain: No
Public Restroom: No
Cross Streets: One

Link Runs
@ Saratoga & Kalia: Saratoga & Beachwalk

Comment: Fort DeRussy is an open but active US military installation. The property was purchased by the US Army in 1904 from the first Chinese millionaire in Hawaii. The Hawaii Army Museum is on the ocean side of Kalia Road. It is free and open to the public.

# Warrior
## Fort DeRussy Loop

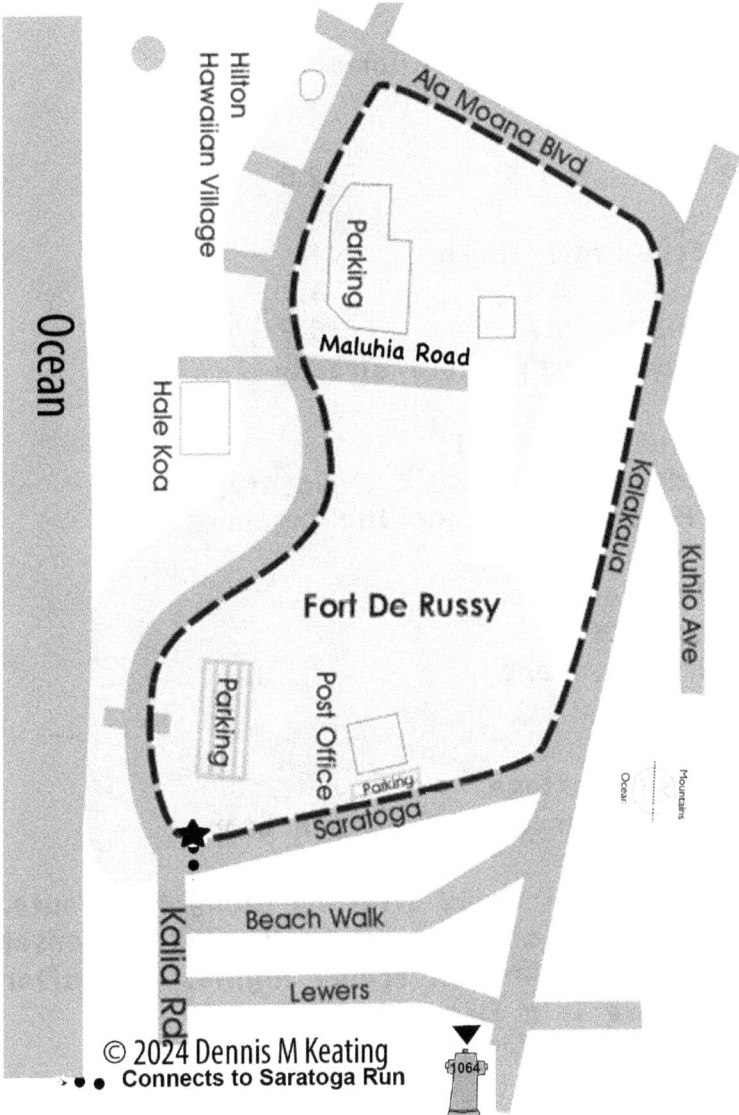

Ocean

Hilton Hawaiian Village

Ala Moana Blvd

Parking

Maluhia Road

Hale Koa

Kalakaua

Kuhio Ave

Fort De Russy

Parking

Post Office

Parking

Saratoga

Ocean ⋯⋯ Mountains

Beach Walk

Kalia Rd

Lewers

1064

© 2024 Dennis M Keating
Connects to Saratoga Run

# Strolling
## A Beachfront Loop

Miles   Kilometers

Balloon on
String Loop    1.3        2.0

Round Trip Start/Finish
@ 1064         2.4        3.9
@ The Wall    3.7         5.9
@ Rainbow    You're here already

Scene: The beachfront
Start: Edge of Beachwalk @ Saratoga
Return Point: None. Loop the lagoon

Water Fountain: Yes
Restroom: Yes
Cross Streets: None

Link Runs
@ Edge of Saratoga
@ Bridge at far side of Lagoon Loop

Comment: Tourist enjoy strolling along this route. You can catch a drink, a meal, and a sunset after your run. And on Friday nights, just after sunset, there is a fireworks show.

# Strolling

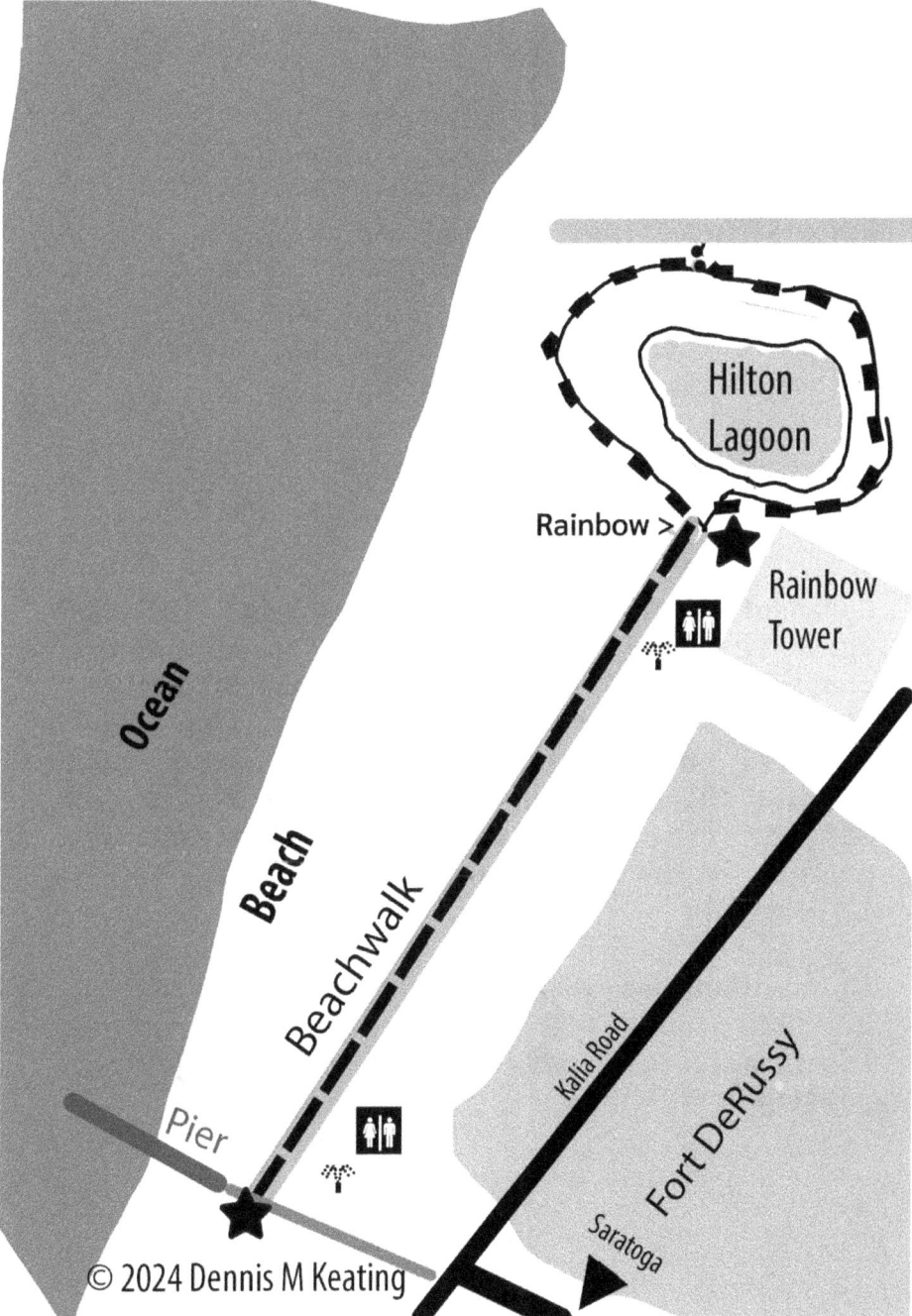

Ocean

Hilton Lagoon

Rainbow >

Rainbow Tower

Beach

Beachwalk

Kalia Road

Fort DeRussy

Pier

Saratoga

© 2024 Dennis M Keating

# Strolling Part 1
## The Beachwalk portion of Strolling

Miles  Kilometers

|            | Miles | Kilometers |
|------------|-------|------------|
| One Way    | .4    | .7         |
| Round Trip | .9    | 1.4        |

Scene: The beachfront
Start: Edge of Saratoga
Return Point: Rainbow

Water Fountain: Yes
Restroom: Yes
Cross Streets: None

Comment: Please view the Strolling page for Link Runs. While Strolling is a short route, we are choosing to provide a more detailed breakdown. We do this for several reasons. We have observed many visiting casual runners and newbies choose to run only Part 1 or Part 2 and not the other. Also, as the Rainbow starting point is in the middle of this route, we want to highlight it.

In addition, we wish to welcome and encourage all newcomers> We offer these two attractive short routes as a way of saying, "Come join us. Jogging is fun."

# Strolling Part 1
## Beachwalk Strip

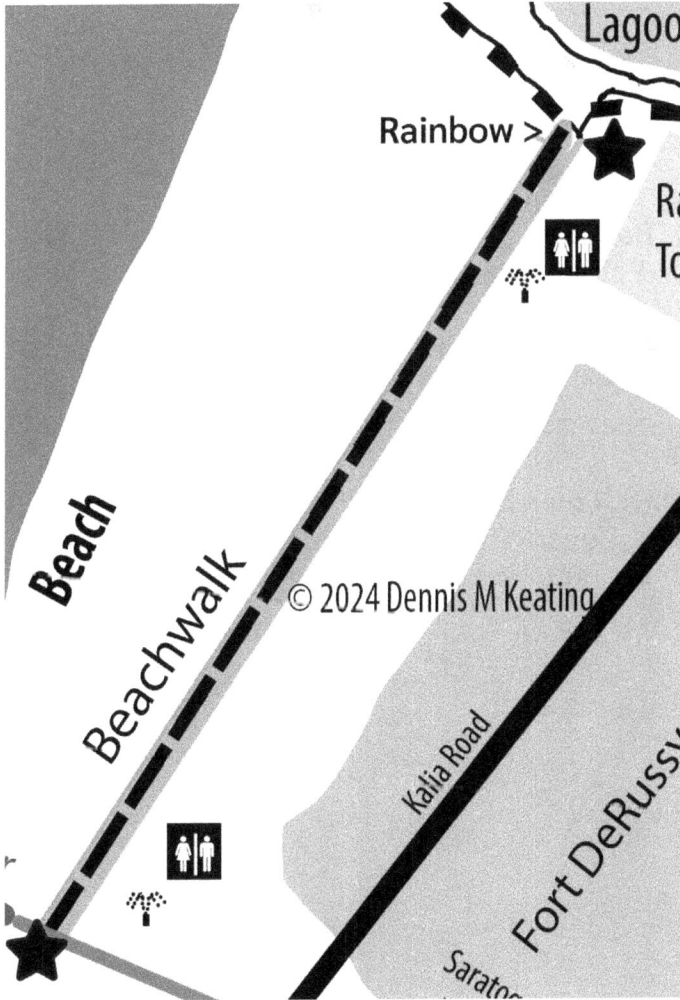

Lagoo

Rainbow >

Ra
To

Beach

Beachwalk

© 2024 Dennis M Keating

Kalia Road

Fort DeRussv

Sarato

# Strolling Part 2
## The Lagoon portion of Strolling

Miles  Kilometers

Lagoon Loop        .4        .6

Scene: The Lagoon
Start: Rainbow
Return Point: None. Loop the lagoon

Water Fountain: No
Restroom: No
Cross Streets: None

Comment: Comment: Please view the Strolling page for Link Runs. This is a short run for newcomers to, as we say in Honolulu, get their feet wet,

# Strolling Part 2
## The Lagoon

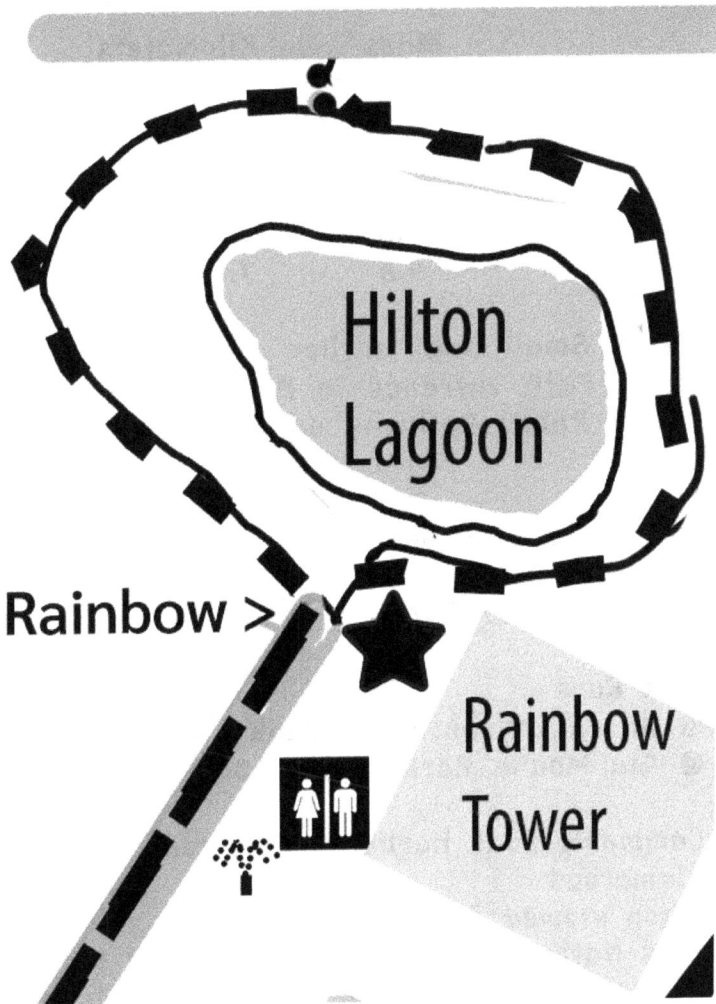

Hilton
Lagoon

Rainbow >

Rainbow
Tower

# A Bridge not too far
## A connector Route

|              | Miles | Kilometers |
|--------------|-------|------------|
| One Way      | .6    | .9         |

Round Trip Start/Finish
| @ Rainbow | 1.6 | 2.7 |
| @ 1064    | 3.6 | 5.8 |
| @ Walls   | 4.8 | 7.8 |

Scene: Small boat harbor
Start: Path entrance to the Hilton Lagoon
Return Point: Pathway entrance to Ala Moana Park

Water Fountain: No
Restroom: No
Cross Streets: Two

Link Runs
@ Hilton Lagoon: Beachwalk
@ Ala Moana Park: Going Local & Park Combo

Comment: Boat harbors often tend to be more glamorous
when viewed from a distance.
Side Note: Be attentive to roadway traffic, Joggers are uncommon creatures in harbor areas.

# A Bridge not too far

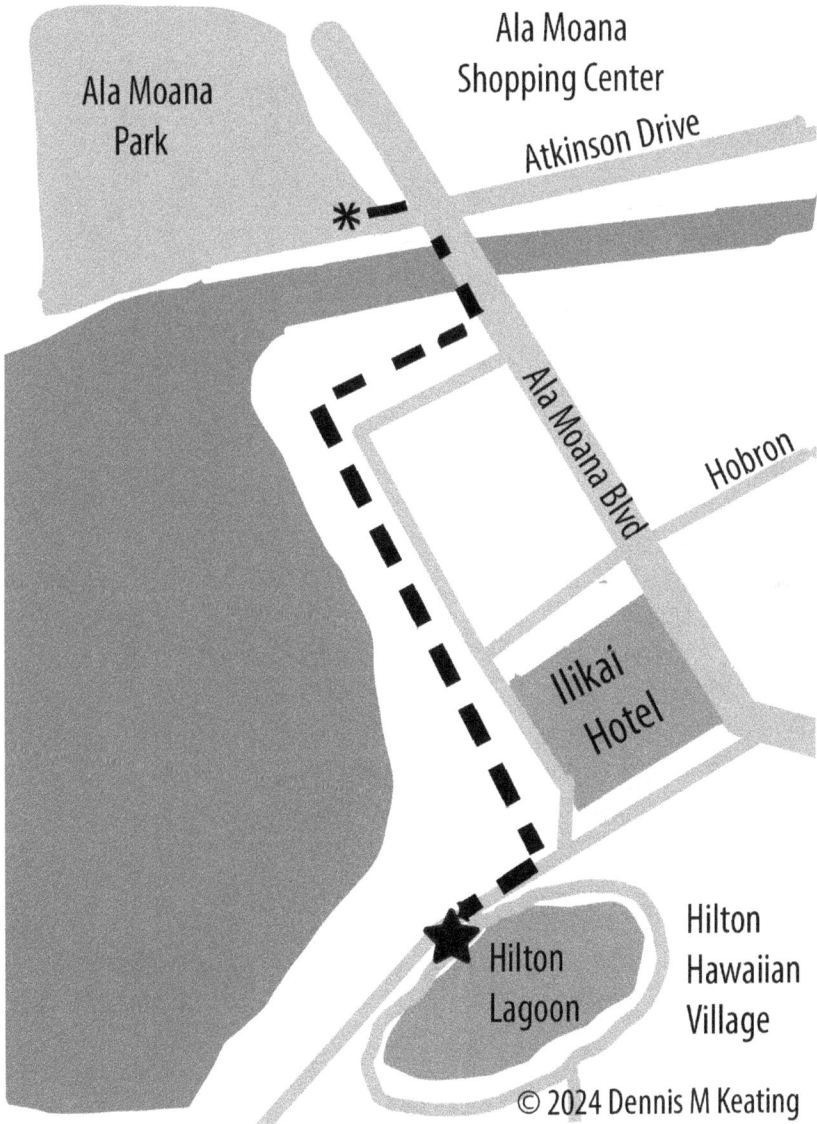

Ala Moana Park

Ala Moana Shopping Center

Atkinson Drive

＊

Ala Moana Blvd

Hobron

Ilikai Hotel

Hilton Lagoon

Hilton Hawaiian Village

© 2024 Dennis M Keating

41

# Going Local
## Ala Moana Park

|  | Miles | Kilometers |
|---|---|---|
| One Loop | 1.9 | 3.0 |

**Up & Back if Start/Finish**

| | | |
|---|---|---|
| @ 1064 | 5.4 | 8.7 |
| @ Walls | 6.7 | 10.8 |
| @ Rainbow | 3.5 | 5.6 |

Scene: A popular local park
Start: Park entrance on Waikiki side
Return Point: None. A loop run

Water Fountain: Yes
Restroom: Yes
Cross Streets: Two

Link Runs
@ Park Entrance: Bridge
@ Magic Island: Green Flash
@ Boat Harbor End: Owl & Nun

Comment: Ala Moana Park is Honolulu's playground. While visitors enjoy Waikiki, locals favor Ala Moana Park. It's our place to swim, jog, play and hold all kinds of family get togethers.

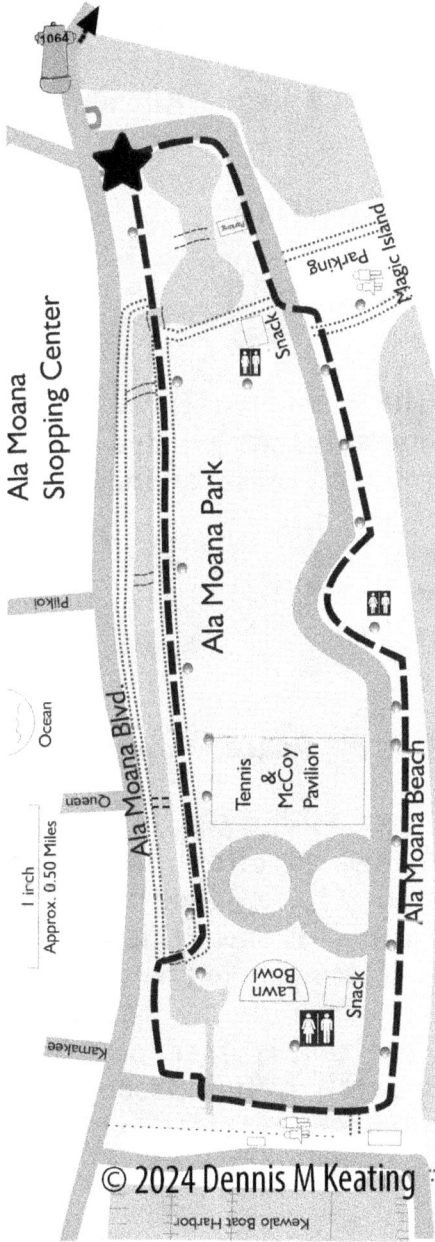

# Going Local

Ala Moana
Shopping Center

Ala Moana Park

Ala Moana Beach

Magic Island

Parking

Tennis
&
McCoy
Pavilion

Lawn
Bowl

Snack

Snack

Ala Moana Blvd

Ocean

Pi'ikoi

Queen

Kamakee

Magic Island

Kewalo Boat Harbor

1 inch
Approx. 0.50 Miles

1064

© 2024 Dennis M Keating

# The Green Flash
## Magic Island

|                      | Miles | Kilometers |
|----------------------|-------|------------|
| Entrance & Loop      | 1.0   | 1.6        |

Up & Back if Start/Finish

|            | Miles | Kilometers |
|------------|-------|------------|
| @ 1064     | 5.0   | 8.1        |
| @ Walls    | 6.3   | 10.1       |
| @ Rainbow  |       |            |

Scene: View the ocean on three sides
Start: Pathway entrance on downtown side
Return Point: None. Lasso shaped loop

Water Fountain: Yes
Public Restroom: Yes
Cross Streets: None

Link Run
@ Ala Moana Park Route: Going Local

Comment: Magic Island is highly popular with local joggers and strollers. Also, don't let the name fool you. It's a landfill, not an island. However, as landfills go, this one has magical beauty. Late afternoon joggers can stick around for the sun to drop below the horizon. If you do, and the horizon is free of clouds, you may be lucky and catch a two second glimpse of the optical (and almost mythical) phenomenon known as The Green Flash.

# The Green Flash

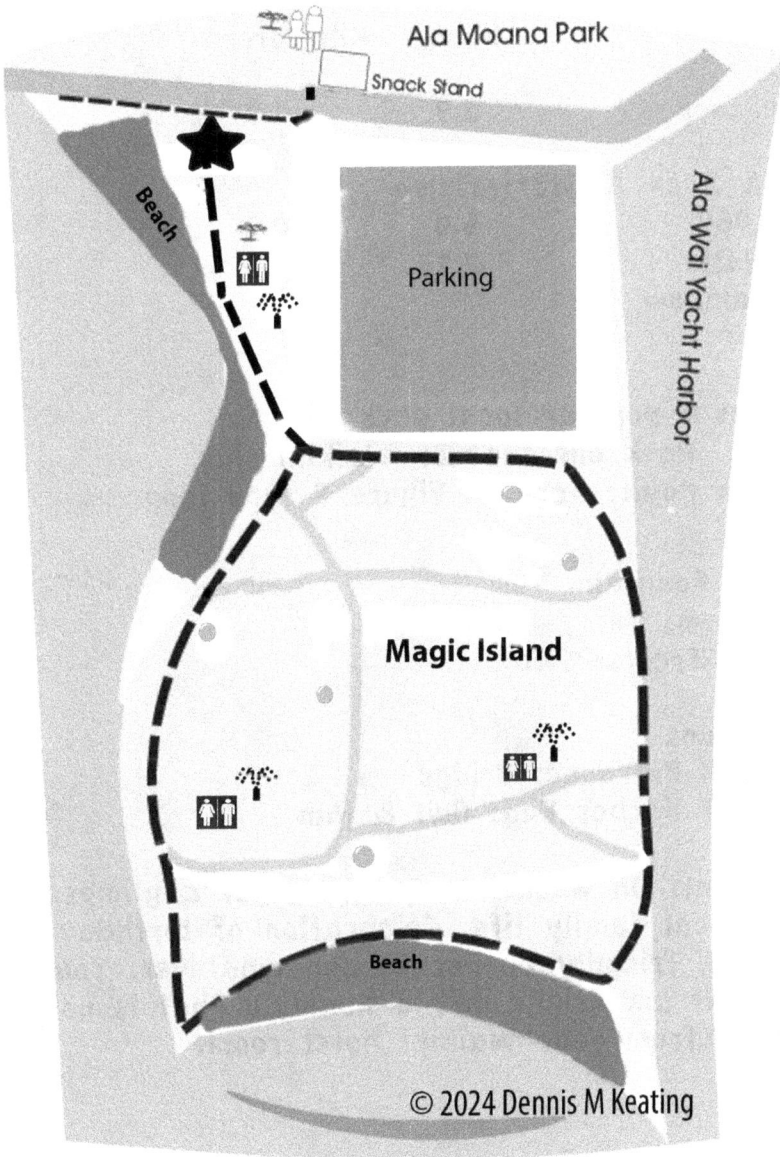

Ala Moana Park

Snack Stand

Beach

Parking

Ala Wai Yacht Harbor

Magic Island

Beach

© 2024 Dennis M Keating

# Da Kine Combo
## Ala Moana Park & Magic Island

|  | Miles | Kilometers |
|---|---|---|
| One Loop | 2.9 | 4.7 |
|  |  |  |
| Up & Back if Start/Finish |  |  |
| @ 1064 | 6.4 | 10.3 |
| @ Walls | 7.7 | 12.3 |
| @ Rainbow |  |  |

Scene: A popular local park
Start: Park entrance on Waikiki side
Return Point: None. A Figure 8 type loop

Water Fountain: Yes
Restroom: Yes
Cross Streets: Two

Link Runs
@ Park Entrance: Bridge
@ Boat Harbor End: Owl & Nun

Comment: On weekends, you can get a glimpse into local family life. Celebration of birthday parties, friendly barbecues and whatever. You will get an insight into a Honolulu that is not visible from your Waikiki hotel room.

# Da Kine Combo

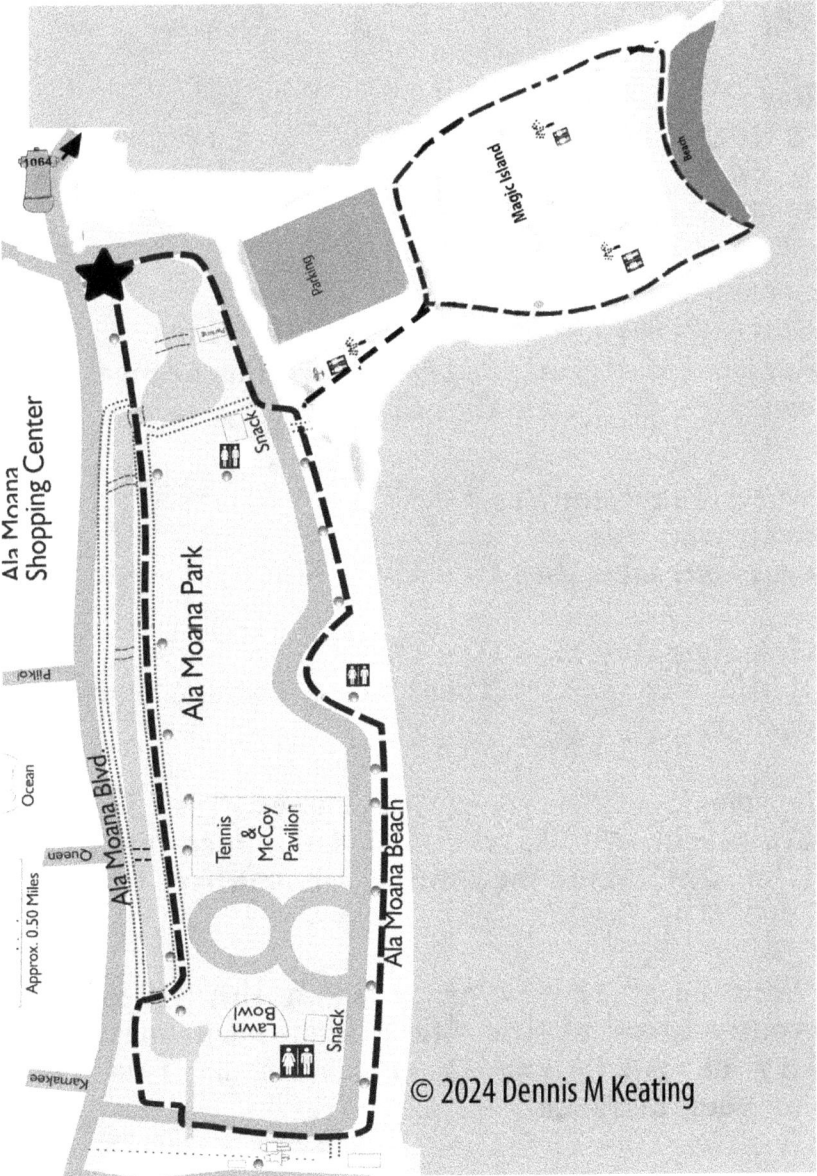

Ala Moana
Shopping Center

Ala Moana Park

Tennis & McCoy Pavilion

Lawn Bowl

Magic Island

Parking

Beach

Snack

Ala Moana Blvd.

Ala Moana Beach

Pllkol

Ocean

Queen

Kamakee

Approx. 0.50 Miles

1064

© 2024 Dennis M Keating

# The Owl & the Nun
## Kewalo Basin Harbor

|  | Miles | Kilometers |
|---|---|---|
| The Owl Loop | .8 | 1.3 |

Round Trip Start/Finish

|  | Miles | Kilometers |
|---|---|---|
| @ 1064 | 5.4 | 8.7 |
| @ Walls | 6.7 | 10.8 |
| @ Rainbow | | |

Scene: Tour boat harbor
Start: Sidewalk at Ala Moana Boulevard
Return Point: Far tip of breakwater beyond the owl

Water Fountain: Yes
Restroom: Yes
Cross Streets: Two

Link Runs
@ Ala Moana Park Loop: Going Local & Park Combo

Comment: This route is named for its two Sculptural Works: the Ano Lani Pueo art piece (The Owl) and the statue of Mother Marianne Cope (The Nun).

Nota Bene: If you are running this route as a continuation of the Ala Moana Park route, add .19 of a mile, or .3 kilometers or 1,000 feet to your distance.

# The Owl & the Nun

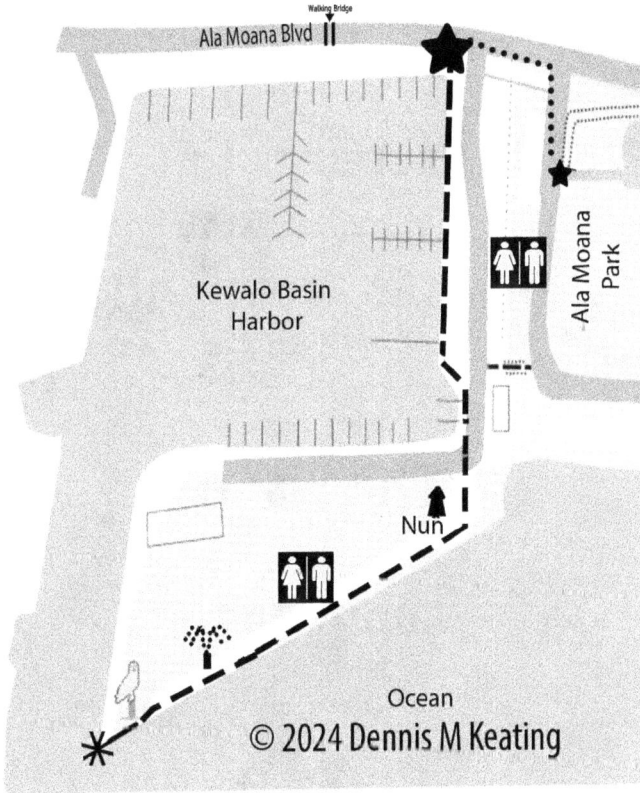

Ala Moana Blvd

Walking Bridge

Kewalo Basin Harbor

Ala Moana Park

Nun

Ocean

© 2024 Dennis M Keating

For this Final Route

Prepare to

Give it your all.

This is a

Long one.

So

# Go

# For

# Broke

# Go For Broke
## The Owl - Gas Station Loop

|  | Miles | Kilometers |
|---|---|---|
| Full Loop | 16.5 | 26.5 |

Route: If you consider a 26.2-mile marathon to be no biggie, this run is for you. It combines several of our runs and goes to the two extreme turn around points in this book.

Start/Finish: 1064, The Wall or anywhere on the route
Turn Around Points: The Gas Station and the Kewalo Basin Breakwater behind the Owl

Water Fountain: Yes
Public Restroom: Yes
Cross Streets: Fifteen

Link Runs
None. You've gone the distance. Congrats.

Comment: "Go for Broke" is a local gambling term that means betting everything on a single card or roll of the dice. During World War II it was the motto of the highly decorated 442 Regimental Combat Team. The 442 and the 100th Infantry Battalion were mainly composed of Hawaii born Nisei (American citizens born to Japanese immigrant parents). At that time, due to the bombing of Pearl Harbor and the imperfect realities of American society, these loyal Americans faced extreme racial discrimination. To prove their love for the Red, White and Blue and show their grit, they chose to Go for Broke!

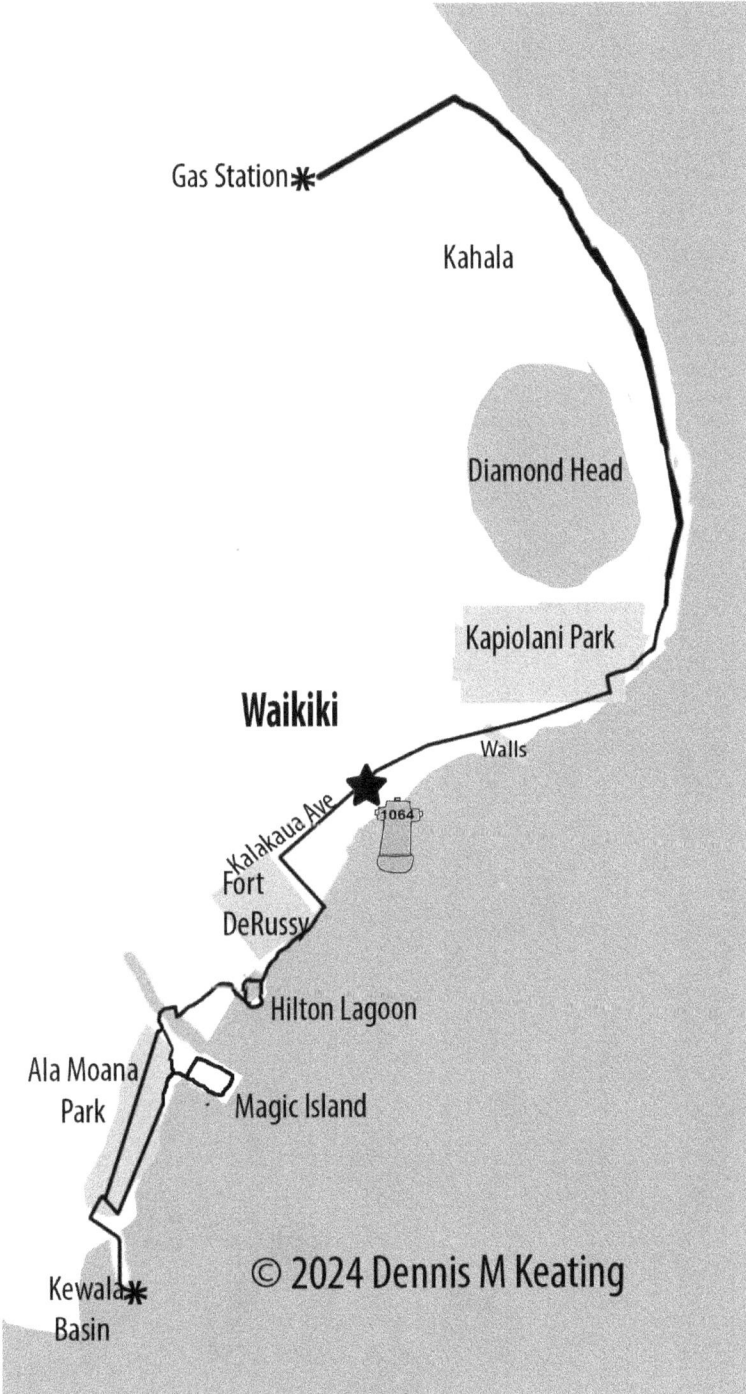

# Go For Broke

Gas Station ✳

Kahala

Diamond Head

Kapiolani Park

**Waikiki**

Walls

Kalakaua Ave

1064

Fort
DeRussy

Hilton Lagoon

Ala Moana
Park

Magic Island

© 2024 Dennis M Keating

Kewala ✳
Basin

# Congrats!

# All Pau!
# (All Finished)

# What's Next?

# That's obvious

The

HONOLULU Marathon

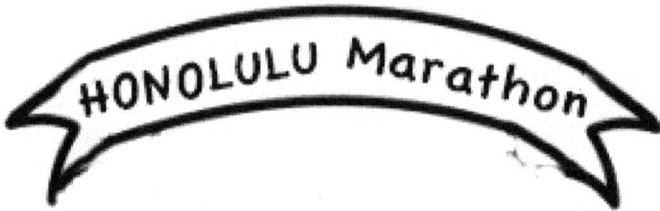

Unsure if you are ready
to run a Marathon?
Then read,

*Can I, should I run a Marathon?*

By Dennis M Keating
Available on Amazon in 2025

Postscript

Keating is a retired, married, mid-eighty-year-old who lives and relaxes in Waikiki.

Keating has worked in 27 countries. Along with living in 8 states, he has kept homes in Germany for twenty years, China for ten years and Thailand for three years. Being an old guy with a peripatetic raconteur's heart, he enjoys good conversations. If you want to chat about running; writing books; Europe; Asia; life in Hawaii; your personal life issues or whatever else you like, including your comments/complaints about this book, and even religion and politics, he is most happy to do it. He is available to meet up on most weekday morning for coffee (your treat) in either Waikiki or by Ala Moana Shopping Center. Feel free to contact him with an invitation to lostpuka@gmail.com. Otherwise, he says get out there and do your jogging thing.

And finally,
You must Remember this
A Jog is not just a Jog.
It's a thing for Health,
Love and Glory.
Like
A Case of Do or Die,
So always try
To do your Best.
The World will
Always welcome Joggers
As time goes by.